Clean
10 DAY GREEN SMOOTHIE CLEANSE PROTEIN COOKBOOK

Clean & Healthy High Protein Recipes to Help You Lose Weight
AFTER 10 Day Green Smoothie Cleanse or Detox Diet

TRISHA MYERS

ISBN-13: 978-1503085671
ISBN-10: 1503085678

Table of Contents

YOU DESERVE PERMANENT WEIGHT LOSS!

Don't become a victim of rebound weight gain after your 10 day smoothie cleanse. Admittedly, regaining weight will be your greatest challenge in all your efforts to ever lose weight. For this reason, maintaining a lower body weight and reducing rebound weight gain will inevitably be your biggest struggle after you've successful lost some weight. But, you can beat this!

It has been scientifically proven that the body tends to regain weight after almost any detox or cleanse program. According to a member of the obesity research team of renowned Obesity Researcher Dr Erik Hemmingsson, rebound often occurs because the body tends to return to its old habits. In an effort to keep things as it used to be, the body then naturally develops a host of defense tactics which are all working together to fight any form of weight loss you've experienced. Some of these common defense tactics include hunger pangs, reduced energy levels, and targeted food cravings.

Nevertheless, you don't have to be disheartened by all this, there is hope. The good news is that there have been proven scientific studies which have all concurred that a high protein diet is necessary for experiencing permanent weight loss. Now, not all high protein diets are created equal. A healthy high protein diet should be well balanced with the right foods combined with the right cooking methods.

This cookbook contains specially crafted recipes which are all geared towards providing a healthy high protein diet to enhance permanent weight loss after a cleanse or detox program. After all, you deserve it! The recipes include a variety of lean protein, unprocessed food, natural whole foods, low sugars and healthy fats. Additionally, the recipes are all developed to help you lose weight after your smoothie or detox cleanse and are based on diet specific guidelines for continued weight loss.

YOU ARE IN CONTROL AGAIN

With this book, Follow-up Protein Cookbook for 10 Day Smoothie Cleanse, you'll be able to take hold of clean, healthy and mouthwatering high protein meals that will help you to maintain your weight loss and even lose more weight. Overall, this protein cookbook will help you to further take hold of your right to experience permanent weight loss and increased longevity.

Whatever recipes you choose from this collection of over 100 high protein recipes, it's totally up to you. All you'll need to do is follow the instructions in this book along with the different methods of preparing and cooking healthy high protein meals. Yes, it can become really easy. In some cases, feel free to make your own diet friendly ingredient substitutions based on your preferences or individual situations.

Now, it's time to try your hand at creating healthy, easy and tasty high protein meals with these specially created recipes.

Enjoy every bite, while you experience permanent weight loss!

PROTEIN BREAKFAST RECIPES

Baked Spinach Omelet

This is a great and incredibly delicious way to prepare an omelet for breakfast when having company. Only two steps are needed with this recipe to prepare these delicious omelets.

MAKES: 2 servings
PREPARATION TIME: 10 minutes
COOKING TIME: 17 minutes

6 Egg Whites
Sea Salt, to taste
Freshly Ground Black Pepper, to taste
¾ cup scallions, chopped
1 cup Fresh Spinach, chopped finely
6-8 Cherry Tomatoes, sliced

Directions:

1. Preheat the oven to 400 degrees F and grease a small baking dish.
2. In a bowl, beat together the egg whites, salt and black pepper. Stir in the scallions and spinach. Transfer the mixture into the prepared baking dish.
3. Place tomato slices on top, pressing gently. Bake for about 17 minutes.

Spiced Pumpkin Oatmeal

This warm and creamy bowl of spiced pumpkin oatmeal is a great way to start your morning. The Egg whites gives added proteins into this healthy grain meal.

MAKES: 4 servings
PREPARATION TIME: 10 minutes
COOKING TIME: 20 minutes

3 cups Water
Pinch of Sea Salt
1 cup Steel Cut Oats
4 Egg Whites, beaten
½ cup Homemade Pumpkin Puree
½ teaspoon Ground Cinnamon
¼ teaspoon Ground Ginger
¼ teaspoon Ground Nutmeg
Stevia, to taste
¼ cup Almonds, chopped

Directions:

1. In a pan, add the water and salt and bring to a boil. Add the oats and, whilst stirring occasionally, boil for 10 to 15 minutes.
2. Slowly add the egg whites, stirring continuously. Add the pumpkin puree and spices and cook, stirring, for 4 to 5 minutes.
3. Remove from the heat and stir in the stevia. Transfer the oatmeal into serving bowls. Top with almonds and serve.

Chicken Kale Frittata

This recipe makes a super quick, delicious and healthy breakfast for the whole family. This frittata is packed with a healthy dose of egg whites with chicken and kale.

MAKES: 2 servings
PREPARATION TIME: 10 minutes
COOKING TIME: 5 minutes

1 tablespoon Homemade Chicken Broth
1 small Onion, chopped
6 Egg Whites
Sea Salt, to taste
Freshly Ground Black Pepper, to taste
½ cup Cooked Chicken, shredded
1 cup Fresh Kale, trimmed and chopped

Directions:

1. Preheat the grill on a low heat.
2. In an oven proof skillet, heat the broth on a medium heat. Add the onion and cook for 4 to 5 minutes. Meanwhile, in a bowl, beat together the egg whites, salt and black pepper. Stir in the remaining ingredients. Pour the chicken mixture over the onion mixture.
3. Transfer the skillet to the grill and grill for 5 minutes.

Chicken Spinach Muffins

This is a great dish to get your kids to eat healthy vegetables. Chicken and vegetables with egg whites make a perfect combination for these delicious muffins.

MAKES: 4 servings
PREPARATION TIME: 20 minutes
COOKING TIME: 25 minutes

¼ cup Cooked Chicken, chopped
1 cup Fresh Spinach, chopped
1 Red Bell Pepper, seeded and chopped
1 Green Bell Pepper, seeded and chopped
2 Scallions, chopped
⅛ teaspoon Cayenne Pepper
Sea Salt, to taste
Freshly Ground Black Pepper, to taste
12 Egg Whites, beaten

Directions:

1. Preheat the oven to 350 degrees F and grease a 12 cup muffin tray.
2. In a large bowl, mix together the chicken, vegetables, cayenne, salt and black pepper. Place the vegetable mixture in the prepared muffin cups. Evenly pour the egg whites over the vegetable mixture.
3. Bake for 20 to 25 minutes, or until the egg whites are cooked.

Overnight Oatmeal Strawberries

This recipe presents one of the easiest ways to make steel cut oats. These oats are dense, rich, and very filling for a healthy and fantastic breakfast.

MAKES: 2 servings
PREPARATION TIME: 15 minutes (plus time to refrigerate overnight)
COOKING TIME: 30 seconds

1½ cups Almond Milk, unsweetened
1 cup Steel Cut Oats
1 tablespoon Applesauce, unsweetened
1 cup Fresh Strawberries, hulled and sliced
½ teaspoon lemon zest, freshly grated
Pinch of Ground Cinnamon

Directions:

1. In a bowl, mix together 1 cup of almond milk, oats and applesauce. Cover and refrigerate for overnight.
2. Remove from the refrigerator. Transfer the oat mixture into a microwave safe bowl. Stir in the remaining almond milk and microwave for 30 seconds.
3. Transfer into serving bowls. Top with strawberries and lemon zest. Dust with cinnamon and serve.

Oatmeal Stuffed Squash

This recipe is a lovely and fun-loving way to enjoy a breakfast. Also, the spices used in this squash dish gives this breakfast meal a wonderful flavoring.

MAKES: 2 servings
PREPARATION TIME: 10 minutes
COOKING TIME: 40 minutes

1 Acorn Squash, halved and seeded
1½ cups Water
½ cup Steel Cut Oats
1 teaspoon Ground Cinnamon
Pinch of Ground Nutmeg
Pinch of Ground Ginger
Pinch of Sea Salt
2 tablespoons Natural Peanut Butter

Directions:

1. Preheat the oven to 350 degrees F and grease a baking sheet. Place the squash, cut side up, on the prepared baking sheet. Roast until the squash is tender, for about 30 to 35 minutes.
2. Meanwhile, in a microwave safe bowl, add the water and oats. Microwave on high for about 5 minutes. Stir well and microwave for 5 minutes more. Set aside for 5 minutes before stirring in the spices.
3. Fill the acorn squash halves with the oatmeal mixture. Bake for a further 5 minutes, or until the top becomes

golden brown.
4. Arrange the baked squash halves on serving plates. Top with peanut butter and serve.

Morning Berry Bread

We all know that there are some mornings when a quick and healthy breakfast may be just what we need. This is a quick and easy breakfast recipe with the added benefits of healthy nutrients. Fresh berries add a nice flavor to the buttered slices.

MAKES: 2 servings
PREPARATION TIME: 10 minutes

---

2 Whole Wheat Bread Slices, toasted
¼ cup Natural Peanut Butter
1 cup mixed Fresh Berries (for example blueberries, blackberries and/or raspberries)
⅛ teaspoon Ground Cinnamon

Directions:

1. Evenly spread the peanut butter on each slice of bread.
2. Top with berries. Dust with cinnamon and serve.

Seed & Nut Porridge

This is a nourishing super food breakfast with an abundance of healthy nutrients. Fresh strawberries and nuts jazz the flavor of this seed porridge nicely.

MAKES: 2 servings
PREPARATION TIME: 15 minutes (plus time to refrigerate overnight)

---

2 cups Almond Milk, unsweetened
⅓ cup Chia Seeds
3-4 drops Liquid Stevia
½ teaspoon Ground Cinnamon
¼ teaspoon Ground Nutmeg
¼ teaspoon Ground Cardamom
½ cup Fresh Strawberries, hulled and sliced
2 tablespoons Walnuts, chopped

Directions:

1. In a bowl, mix together the almond milk and chia seeds. Stir in the stevia and spices. Cover and refrigerate overnight.
2. Top with the strawberries and walnuts before serving.

Raspberry Quinoa

This is another easy and healthy recipe to start the day with. This quinoa dish is delicious enough that even your kids will love this breakfast.

MAKES: 2 servings
PREPARATION TIME: 10 minutes
COOKING TIME: 15 minutes

2 cups Water
1 cup Quinoa
1 teaspoon Almond Butter
⅔ cup Almond Milk, unsweetened
Stevia, to taste
½ teaspoon Ground Cinnamon
1 cup Fresh Raspberries

Directions:

1. In a pan, add the water and quinoa and bring to the boil on a medium heat. Reduce the heat to low. Cover and simmer for about 15 minutes. Turn off the heat. Keep the pan covered for at least 5 minutes.
2. Stir in the butter, milk, stevia and cinnamon.
3. Transfer the quinoa into serving bowls. Garnish with raspberries before serving.

Spiced Egg Quinoa

This is a delicious and healthy breakfast recipe. This creamy breakfast quinoa is packed with the aromatic blend of spices and the flavors of fresh cranberries.

MAKES: 2 servings
PREPARATION TIME: 10 minutes
COOKING TIME: 30 minutes

½ cup Quinoa
2 cups Almond Milk, unsweetened
½ teaspoon Ground Cinnamon
⅛ teaspoon Ground Ginger
Pinch of Ground Cardamom
Pinch of Ground Nutmeg
Pinch of Sea Salt
Stevia, to taste
1 large Egg White
¼ cup Fresh Cranberries

Directions:

1. Heat a non-stick pan on a medium-high heat. Add the quinoa and cook, stirring continuously for about 2 to 3 minutes. Add the milk and spices and bring to the boil. Reduce the heat to low. Simmer, stirring often, for about 20 to 25 minutes. Remove from the heat and stir in the stevia.
2. In a small bowl, add 2 tablespoon of the cooked quinoa and egg white, and beat until it is well combined. Return

the egg white mixture into the pan on a medium-low heat. Simmer, stirring continuously for 1 to 2 minutes.
3. Transfer the mixture into serving bowls. Top with cranberries and serve.

Nutty Baked Barley

This is a perfect and satisfying breakfast for cold mornings. This nutty and chewy barley is packed with the flavors of fruit, nuts and a hint of cinnamon.

MAKES: 2 servings
PREPARATION TIME: 15 minutes
COOKING TIME: 30 minutes

1½ cups Cooked Barley
¼ cup Almond Milk, unsweetened
2 Egg Whites, beaten
Liquid Stevia, to taste
½ teaspoon Ground Cinnamon
Pinch of Sea Salt
2 tablespoons Walnuts, chopped
½ cup Fresh Raspberries, halved and divided

Directions:

1. Preheat the oven to 350 degrees F and grease a small casserole dish.
2. In a large bowl, except for the raspberries, mix together all of the ingredients. Fold in half of the raspberries. Transfer the mixture into the prepared casserole dish and spread the remaining raspberries evenly on top.
3. Bake for about 30 minutes.

Cranberry Rice Bowl

Start your day with this delicious dish. This refreshing lime zest and aromatic cinnamon infused breakfast bowl is packed with wholesome ingredients.

MAKES: 4 servings
PREPARATION TIME: 15 minutes
COOKING TIME: 2 minutes

1 cup Cooked Brown Rice
½ teaspoon Lime Zest, freshly grated
1 tablespoon Coconut Oil, melted
1 teaspoon Ground Cinnamon
Pinch of Sea Salt
⅓ cup Rice Milk, unsweetened
Stevia, to taste
1 cup Fresh Cranberries

Directions:

1. In a bowl, mix together the cooked rice, lime zest, oil, cinnamon and salt. Transfer the mixture into serving bowls.
2. In a small pan, add the milk and bring to the boil for 1 to 2 minutes. Remove from the heat and stir in the stevia.
3. Evenly pour the milk over the rice mixture. Garnish with cranberries and serve.

SALAD & MEATLESS RECIPES

Fresh Berry Salad

There will be nothing better than this fresh, healthy and delicious mixed berry salad for the whole family.

MAKES: 4 servings
PREPARATION TIME: 20 minutes

1 tablespoon Fresh Lime juice
½ tablespoon Lime Zest, freshly grated
2 tablespoons finely diced Fresh Mint Leaves
Pinch of Sea Salt
2 cups Fresh Strawberries, hulled and sliced
1 cup Fresh Raspberries
1 cup Fresh Blueberries
1 cup Fresh Blackberries
2 tablespoons Fresh Whole Mint Leaves

1. In a small bowl, mix together the lime juice, zest, mint

and salt.
2. Place the mixed berries in a large serving bowl. Add the mint mixture and mix together.
3. Garnish with mint leaves and serve.

Avocado Fruit Salad

Luscious berries combined with a creamy avocado make a wonderfully healthy, refreshing and a delicious fruit salad.

MAKES: 2 servings
PREPARATION TIME: 15 minutes

1 ripe Avocado, peeled, pitted and cubed
1½ cups Fresh Blackberries
1½ cups Fresh Blueberries
2 tablespoons Fresh Lemon juice
½ teaspoon Lemon Zest, freshly grated
Liquid Stevia, to taste

Directions:

1. Gently mix together all of the ingredients in a large serving bowl.
2. Serve immediately.

Spinberry Salad

This is a vibrant spring salad, bursting with the flavors of fresh berries and spinach. The salad ingredients combine with the vinaigrette nicely in this recipe.

MAKES: 2 servings
PREPARATION TIME: 15 minutes

For Salad:
2 cups Fresh Baby Spinach
1 cup Fresh Raspberries
1 cup Fresh Strawberries, hulled and sliced
1 cup cabbage, shredded
½ Red Onion, chopped

For Vinaigrette:
1 small Garlic Clove, minced
1 tablespoon finely diced Fresh Cilantro Leaves
2 tablespoons Apple Cider Vinegar
2 tablespoons Olive Oil
2 tablespoons Fresh Lemon juice
Sea Salt, to taste
Freshly Ground Black Pepper, to taste

Directions:

1. Mix together all of the salad ingredients in a large bowl.
2. In a small bowl, add the vinaigrette ingredients and beat until well combined.

3. Pour the vinaigrette over the salad and toss to coat well before serving.

Fresh Green Salad

This green salad is filled with the flavors of fresh garden vegetables. This recipe will help you to make one of the most refreshing, light and delicious salads.

MAKES: 2 servings
PREPARATION TIME: 15 minutes
COOKING TIME: 3 minutes

For Salad:
½ cup Green Beans, sliced into 2-inch pieces
½ cup Green Cabbage, shredded
¼ cup Green Bell Pepper, seeded and sliced thinly
¼ cup Cucumber, seeded and chopped
¼ cup Scallion (green part), chopped
2 cups Iceberg Lettuce, torn

For Vinaigrette
2 tablespoons Apple Cider Vinegar
1 Garlic Clove, minced
½ Jalapeño Pepper, seeded and minced
Sea Salt, to taste
Freshly Ground Black Pepper, to taste

Directions:

1. Place the beans into a pan of boiling water and boil for 3 minutes. Once cooked drain the water from the beans.
2. In a large bowl, mix together all of the salad ingredients.

3. In a small bowl, add the vinaigrette ingredients and beat until well combined.
4. Pour the vinaigrette over the green salad and toss to coat well.
5. Cover and refrigerate to chill before serving.

Vegetable Salad with Eggs

This fresh and tasty salad is a wonderful and healthy combination of vegetables with egg whites and walnuts. This dish is also a great source of healthy nutrients.

MAKES: 2 servings
PREPARATION TIME: 20 minutes

1 cup Broccoli Florets, chopped
2 cups Baby Arugula, chopped
½ cup Fresh Cherry Tomatoes, halved
½ Red Onion, chopped
4 Hard Boiled Eggs, whites separated and chopped
1 tablespoon Fresh Lime juice
Sea Salt, to taste
Freshly Ground Black Pepper, to taste
2 tablespoons Walnuts, chopped

Directions:

1. In a large serving bowl, except for the walnuts, mix together all of the ingredients.
2. Top with walnuts and serve.

Mixed Bean Fiesta

Mix beans and spinach, with this tangy vinaigrette, combines to make a flavorful, light and a fulfilling salad.

MAKES: 4 servings
PREPARATION TIME: 10 minutes

For Salad:
1 cup Cooked White Beans
1 cup Cooked Black Beans
5 cups Baby Spinach
1 medium peeled Ripe Avocado, pitted and cubed

For Vinaigrette:
1 Garlic Clove, minced
2 tablespoons Apple Cider Vinegar
3 tablespoons Olive Oil
2 tablespoons Fresh Lemon juice
Sea Salt, to taste
Freshly Ground Black Pepper, to taste

Directions:

1. In a large bowl, mix together all of the salad ingredients.
2. In a small bowl, add the vinaigrette ingredients and beat until well combined.
3. Pour the vinaigrette over the salad and toss to coat well.

Quinoa with Green Beans

This recipe combines protein-rich quinoa and crunchy green beans to make an incredibly delicious and nutritional vegetarian meal.

MAKES: 4 servings
PREPARATION TIME: 15 minutes
COOKING TIME: 20 minutes

2 cups Fresh Green Beans, trimmed and halved
2 Garlic Cloves, minced
3 tablespoons Olive Oil
Sea Salt, to taste
Freshly Ground Black Pepper, to taste
2 cups Homemade Vegetable Broth
1 cup Red Quinoa, soaked and rinsed
3 Scallions, sliced thinly
3 tablespoons Fresh Lime juice
1 teaspoon Lime Zest, freshly grated
½ cup Walnuts, chopped

Directions:

1. Preheat the oven to 425 degrees F. In a bowl, mix together the beans, garlic, 1 tablespoon of oil, salt and black pepper, and toss to coat well. Transfer the bean mixture into a baking dish and roast for 15 to 20 minutes.
2. Add the broth to a pan and bring to a boil on a medium heat. Add the quinoa and return the broth to the boil

before reducing the heat to low. Simmer, covered, for about 15 minutes before removing the pan from the heat. Let it cool.

3. In a large serving bowl, mix together the beans, quinoa and scallions. Drizzle with the remaining lime juice and oil, and season with salt and black pepper.

4. Top with lime zest and walnuts before serving.

Wild Rice & Asparagus Pilaf

This substantial wild rice pilaf is easy to prepare, delicious, and is a great vegetarian dish that is also perfect as an entrée for potlucks.

MAKES: 4 servings
PREPARATION TIME: 15 minutes
COOKING TIME: 55 minutes

2½ cups Homemade Vegetable Broth
1 cup Wild Rice
1 tablespoon Olive Oil
Sea Salt, to taste
Freshly Ground Black Pepper, to taste
½ cup Fresh Asparagus, trimmed and cut into 2-inch pieces
¼ cup Cashew nuts, chopped
1 tablespoon Fresh Lemon juice

Directions:

1. In a pan of boiling water, add the asparagus and cook for 4 to 5 minutes. Drain the water from the pan and set aside.
2. Add the broth to a pan and bring to a boil on a medium heat. Add the rice, oil, salt and black pepper and return the broth to the boil. Reduce the heat, cover, and simmer for 45 minutes.
3. Stir in the asparagus, cashew nuts and lemon juice, and simmer for a further 5 minutes. Turn off the heat and keep the pan covered for at least 10 minutes. With a fork, fluff the rice.

4. Serve warm.

Grilled Vegetable Combo

This is a perfect and versatile recipe uses several vegetables to deliver a hearty bowl. The marinade adds a wonderfully delicious and tangy taste to the vegetables.

MAKES: 4 servings
PREPARATION TIME: 20 minutes
COOKING TIME: 10 minutes

1 medium Eggplant, cut into ½-inch round slices
1 medium Yellow Squash, cut into ½-inch round slices
1 medium Zucchini, cut into ½-inch round slices
2 Plum Tomatoes, sliced into 4 pieces
2 Garlic Cloves, minced
½ cup Fresh Rosemary, minced
2 tablespoons Fresh Lemon Juice
3 tablespoons Olive Oil
2 tablespoons Apple Cider Vinegar
¼ teaspoon Cayenne Pepper
Sea Salt, to taste
Freshly Ground Black Pepper, to taste

Directions:

1. Preheat the grill to a medium-high heat. Grease the grill grate.
2. In a large bowl, add all of the vegetables. In a small bowl, add the remaining ingredients and beat until combined. Add the oil mixture into the bowl with the vegetables.

Toss to coat well and set aside for at least 5 minutes.
3. Place the vegetables on the grill. Cook for 10 minutes, flipping after 5 minutes.

Mixed Bean Patties

These vegetarian bean patties are flavorful, delicious and delightfully healthy.

MAKES: 4 servings
PREPARATION TIME: 15 minutes
COOKING TIME: 20 minutes

---

1 cup Cooked Garbanzo Beans, mashed
1 cup Cooked Black Beans, mashed
1 small Onion, chopped finely
1 Garlic Clove, minced
½ teaspoon Dried Thyme, crushed
2 tablespoons Fresh Thyme, chopped
1 Egg White
Sea Salt, to taste
Freshly Ground Black Pepper, to taste

Directions:

1. Preheat the oven to 425 degrees F and line a baking sheet with parchment paper.
2. In a large bowl mix together all of the ingredients. Make your desired sized patties from the mixture.
3. Arrange the patties on the prepared baking sheet. Bake the patties for 10 minutes on each side.

Baked Tofu with Sauce

This recipe makes a simple yet magical dish of delicious and nutrient chocked baked tofu. You will find the tofu to be perfectly baked in a flavorful sauce.

MAKES: 4 servings
PREPARATION TIME: 10 minutes
COOKING TIME: 30 minutes

2 tablespoons Fresh Lime juice
2 tablespoons Tamari
1 teaspoon Olive Oil
1 (12-ounce) package Extra Firm Tofu, pressed and cut into 8 slices

Directions:

1. Preheat the oven to 350 degrees F and grease a baking pan.
2. In a small bowl, mix together the lime juice, tamari and oil. Arrange the tofu slices on the prepared baking dish in a single layer. Evenly pour the lime juice mixture over the tofu slices.
3. Bake for 25 to 30 minutes. Serve warm.

Spiced Lentil Stew

A hearty and filling stew prepared in a pressure cooker. This simple lentil stew is not only hearty and delicious but also rich in healthy nutrients.

MAKES: 4 servings
PREPARATION TIME: 10 minutes
COOKING TIME: 45 minutes

2 cups Red Lentils
8 cups Water
⅓ cup Olive Oil
1 medium Onion, chopped
2-3 Garlic Cloves, minced
1 teaspoon Fresh Ginger, minced
2 Plum Tomatoes, chopped finely
¼ cup Fresh Parsley, chopped
½ teaspoon Cayenne Pepper
⅛ teaspoon Ground Turmeric
Sea Salt, to taste
Freshly Ground Black Pepper, to taste

Directions:

1. In a pressure cooker, add all of the ingredients and bring to a boil on a high heat.
2. Reduce the heat to medium. Cover and cook for 40 to 45 minutes.

FISH & SEAFOOD RECIPES

Bell Pepper Cod

*This hearty cod and bell pepper stew is rich with
wonderfully delicious flavors.*

MAKES: 2 servings
PREPARATION TIME: 15 minutes
COOKING TIME: 25 minutes

*½ pound Cod Fillets
1 Onion, sliced
1 Garlic Clove, minced
¼ cup Tomatoes, crushed
1 teaspoon Capers
¼ cup Green Bell Pepper, seeded and chopped
¼ cup Red Bell Pepper, seeded and chopped
¼ cup Olive Oil
⅓ cup Homemade Fish Broth
Sea Salt, to taste
Freshly Ground Black Pepper, to taste
2 Hard Boiled Eggs, whites separated and sliced
2 tablespoons Fresh Lime juice*

Directions:

1. In a large pan, except for the egg whites and lime juice, add all of the ingredients and bring to the boil on a high heat. Reduce the heat, cover, and simmer for 20 minutes.
2. Stir in the egg whites and lime juice. Simmer the stew for a further 5 minutes.

Flavor House Shrimp

This recipe makes a luscious seafood stew, one that is a filling and a hearty supper for the whole family.

MAKES: 4 servings
PREPARATION TIME: 15 minutes
COOKING TIME: 50 minutes

4 Carrots, peeled and cubed
1 cup Fresh Tomatoes, crushed
4 cups Homemade Fish Broth
2 tablespoons Coconut Oil
¼ teaspoon Cayenne Pepper
1½ pounds Clams, scrubbed
1 pound large Shrimp, peeled and deveined
½ cup Fresh Basil, chopped
1 tablespoon Fresh Lime juice
Sea Salt, to taste
Freshly Ground Black Pepper, to taste

Directions:

1. In a large pan, add the carrots, tomatoes, broth, oil and cayenne pepper and bring to a boil on a high heat. Reduce the heat to medium-low. Cover tightly and cook for 35 to 45 minutes.
2. Uncover and stir in the clams and shrimp. Cook for a further 4 to 5 minutes. Stir in the basil, lime juice, salt and black pepper and serve.

Baked Seafood Stew

This is an outstanding recipe for a deliciously baked seafood stew.
This dish is easy to prepare and rich in flavors.

MAKES: 4 servings
PREPARATION TIME: 20 minutes
COOKING TIME: 45 minutes

---

1 large Onion, sliced thinly
2 Celery Stalks, chopped
4-5 Garlic Cloves, minced
4 (4-ounce) Halibut Fillets
½ pound large Shrimp, peeled and deveined
2 pounds Mussels, scrubbed and de-bearded
6 Plum Tomatoes, chopped
½ cup Capers
2 teaspoons Fresh Thyme, chopped
2 teaspoons Fresh Oregano, chopped
2 cups Homemade Chicken Broth
¼ cup Olive Oil
½ teaspoon Cayenne Pepper
Sea Salt, to taste
Freshly Ground Black Pepper, to taste

Directions:

1. Preheat the oven to350 degrees F.
2. Place the onion, celery and garlic in a casserole dish. Place the fish fillets, shrimp and mussels over the onion.

Spread the tomatoes, capers and herbs over the seafood. Pour in the broth and oil and sprinkle with the spices.

3. Cover and bake for 35 to 45 minutes.

Mussels in Tomato Sauce

If you have had problems in the past with preparing and cooking mussels, then this is a perfect recipe for you. This recipe will help you make a delicious mussel dish which will be a winner with everyone.

MAKES: 4 servings
PREPARATION TIME: 20 minutes
COOKING TIME: 30 minutes

2 cups Homemade Chicken Broth
2½ cups Tomatoes, chopped
3-4 Garlic Cloves, minced
1 White Onion, chopped very finely
1 teaspoon Dried Rosemary, crushed
3 tablespoons Fresh Cilantro, chopped
¼ teaspoon Cayenne Pepper
4 pounds Mussels, scrubbed and de-bearded
Sea Salt, to taste
Freshly Ground Black Pepper, to taste
2 tablespoons Olive Oil

Directions:

1. In a blender, add 1 cup of broth, the tomatoes and garlic and pulse until a paste forms. Transfer the tomato paste into a large pan. Add the remaining broth, onion, herbs and cayenne pepper to the pan and bring to the boil. Reduce the heat, partially cover and, whilst stirring

occasionally, simmer for 20 to 25 minutes.

2. Add the mussels and bring to a boil on a medium heat. Cook for about 3 minutes, or until the mussels open. Transfer the opened mussels into serving plates. Cook the tomato sauce for a further 2 minutes, season with salt and pepper if required.

3. Pour the tomato sauce over the mussels, drizzle with oil and serve.

Roasted Zucchini Sea Bass

This is a wonderfully delicious roasted fish dish. The vinegar and mint mixture adds a nice flavor to the sea bass and zucchini.

MAKES: 4 servings
PREPARATION TIME: 15 minutes
COOKING TIME: 35 minutes

1 large Onion, chopped
2 tablespoons Olive Oil
1 pound Zucchini, cut into ½-inch pieces
4 (6-ounce) Sea Bass Fillets
Sea Salt, to taste
Freshly Ground Black Pepper, to taste
1 tablespoon Apple Cider Vinegar
2 tablespoons finely diced Fresh Mint Leaves

Directions:

1. Preheat the oven to 400 degrees F and grease a baking dish.
2. Place the onion in the baking dish and drizzle with 1 tablespoon of oil. Roast the onion for about 15 minutes, stirring every 5 minutes. Add the zucchini to the baking dish and roast for a further 10 minutes before removing the baking dish from the oven.
3. Increase the temperature of the oven to 450 degrees F. Remove the onion and zucchini from the center of the baking dish. Arrange the fish fillets into the center.

Sprinkle with salt and black pepper and place the vegetables over the fish fillets. Roast for 8 to 10 minutes.

4. In a small bowl, mix together the vinegar and mint. Serve the fish and vegetables with a drizzling of the vinegar mixture.

Baked Lemony Fish

This is a wonderfully delicious recipe for baked fish. The Lemon slices bring a refreshingly zesty touch to the dish, and the chili powder gives the fish fillets a mild spicy kick.

MAKES: 2 servings
PREPARATION TIME: 15 minutes
COOKING TIME: 30 minutes

2 Shallots, sliced thinly
1 Lemon, sliced thinly
¼ cup Fresh Thyme, minced
¼ teaspoon Chili Powder
Sea Salt, to taste
Freshly Ground Black Pepper, to taste
2 (6-ounce) Halibut Fillets

Directions:

1. Preheat the oven to 450 degrees F and grease a baking dish.
2. Place half of the shallots and lemon into the prepared baking dish. Generously sprinkle them with thyme and spices. Arrange the fish fillets over the lemon slices and shallots. Sprinkle with salt and black pepper. Place the remaining lemon slices and shallots over the fish.
3. Bake for 25 to 30 minutes.

Olive Garlic Cod

This recipe makes a quick, super easy and delicious cod dish. This will be a great hit for busy weeknight dinners.

MAKES: 4 servings
PREPARATION TIME: 10 minutes
COOKING TIME: 20 minutes

---

2 Garlic Cloves, minced
¼ teaspoon Cayenne Pepper
Sea Salt, to taste
Freshly Ground Black Pepper, to taste
4 (6-ounce) Cod Fillets
1 tablespoon Olive Oil
2 tablespoons Fresh Lime juice

Directions:

1. Preheat the oven to 400 degrees F and grease a baking dish.
2. In a bowl, mix together the garlic and spices. Add the fillets and generously rub them with the garlic mixture. Place the cod fillets into the prepared baking dish in a single layer. Drizzle with oil and lime juice.
3. Bake for 15 to 20 minutes.

Tomato Baked Sea Bass

This is a tasty sea bass recipe which has lots of nice flavors. The combination of citrus fruit and herbs provides a refreshing and aromatic touch to the sea bass.

MAKES: 4 servings
PREPARATION TIME: 20 minutes
COOKING TIME: 55 minutes

1¼ cups Homemade Chicken Broth
¼ cup Fresh Lemon juice
¼ cup Fresh Lime juice
2 cups Tomatoes, chopped finely
1 large Onion, chopped finely
2 Garlic Cloves, minced
1 tablespoon Fresh Basil, chopped
1 tablespoon Fresh Oregano, chopped
1 tablespoon Fresh Thyme, chopped
½ tablespoon Lemon Zest, freshly grated
½ tablespoon Lime Zest, freshly grated
Sea Salt, to taste
Freshly Ground Black Pepper, to taste
4 (4-ounce) Sea Bass Fillets

Directions:

1. In a skillet, heat 3 tablespoons of the broth. Add the onion and cook, stirring for 3 to 4 minutes. Add the garlic and cook for a further minute. Add the tomatoes and

cook, stirring, for 4 to 5 minutes. Stir in remaining ingredients, except the fish fillets, and bring to the boil. Reduce the heat and, whilst stirring occasionally, simmer for 20 to 25 minutes.

2. Preheat the oven to 375 degrees F and grease a baking dish.

3. Place the fish fillets into the prepared baking dish. Pour the sauce over the fillets and bake until cooked, for approximately15 to 20 minutes.

Baked Salmon Parcel

This recipe provides a lovely combination of salmon with simple ingredients. It is also a healthy and delicious way to eat this fish.

MAKES: 2 servings
PREPARATION TIME: 15 minutes (plus time to marinate)
COOKING TIME: 45 minutes

2 tablespoons Fresh Lemon Juice
1 tablespoon Olive Oil
2 Garlic Cloves, minced
½ tablespoon finely diced Fresh Thyme
½ tablespoon finely diced Fresh Oregano
Sea Salt, to taste
Freshly Ground Black Pepper, to taste
2 (6-ounce) Salmon Fillets

Directions:

1. In a bowl, mix together all of the ingredients, except the salmon. Add the fillets and generously rub with the garlic mixture. Cover and refrigerate to marinate for at least 1 hour, toss occasionally.
2. Preheat the oven to 375 degrees F. Place the salmon fillets over heavy duty aluminum foil. Top with the remaining marinade and wrap the foil paper to completely seal the fish.
3. Arrange the salmon parcels in a baking dish and bake for 35 to 45 minutes.

Rosemary Stuffed Snapper

This recipe infuses the lovely flavors of fresh rosemary and lime into the snapper. This is an easy yet impressive recipe for baked whole fish.

MAKES: 4 servings
PREPARATION TIME: 15 minutes (plus time to marinate)
COOKING TIME: 45 minutes

1 (2-pound) cleaned and scaled Whole Red Snapper
1 tablespoon Fresh Lime juice
2 tablespoons Coconut Oil, melted
½ teaspoon Cayenne Pepper
Sea Salt, to taste
Freshly Ground Black Pepper, to taste
4-6 Fresh Rosemary Sprigs
4-6 Lime Slices

Directions:

1. Place the snapper on a greased large piece of heavy-duty aluminum foil. Drizzle the cavity of the fish with lime juice and oil. Sprinkle the cavity and outer side of the fish with the spices. Stuff the cavity with the rosemary sprigs and wrap the foil paper to completely seal the fish. Refrigerate to marinate for 8 to 10 hours.
2. Preheat the oven to 350 degrees F. Arrange the parcel on a baking sheet and bake for about 45 minutes.

Vegetable Baked Halibut

This recipe provides a moist and tender baked fish. This super quick and easy to assemble dish is ideal for busy weekdays.

MAKES: 4 servings
PREPARATION TIME: 15 minutes
COOKING TIME: 15 minutes

¼ cup Tamari
¼ cup Fresh Lemon Juice
2 Garlic Cloves, minced
½ tablespoon Fresh Ginger, minced
1 Jalapeño, minced
4 (6-ounce) Haddock Fillets
1 cup Cabbage, shredded
1 cup Green Bell Pepper, seeded and sliced thinly
1 cup Red Bell Pepper, seeded and sliced thinly
¼ cup Scallions, sliced thinly

Directions:

1. Preheat the oven to 425 degrees F.
2. In a bowl, mix together the tamari, lemon juice, garlic, ginger and jalapeño. Add the fish fillets and coat generously. Set aside for 10 minutes.
3. In a bowl, mix together all of the vegetables. Place 4 heavy-duty aluminum foil sheets onto a smooth surface and evenly place the vegetable mixture over the foil sheets. Arrange the fish fillets over the vegetables and drizzle with the remaining ginger mixture.
4. Fold the foil to seal the packet around fish and

vegetables. Bake for 13 to 15 minutes.

Steamed Halibut

This recipe provides a healthy way to cook a fish. Fresh rosemary, garlic and tamari provide the main flavors to this delicious halibut dish.

MAKES: 2 servings
PREPARATION TIME: 15 minutes
COOKING TIME: 20 minutes

2 Scallions, sliced into 3-inch pieces
4 large Cabbage Leaves
2 (6-ounce) Halibut Fillets
2 large Garlic Cloves, minced
½ tablespoon Fresh Rosemary, minced
¼ teaspoon Cayenne Pepper
Sea Salt, to taste
Freshly Ground Black Pepper, to taste
2 tablespoons Water
3 tablespoons Tamari

Directions:

1. Place half of the scallions and the cabbage into a steamer basket. Arrange the fish fillets over the cabbage. Sprinkle with garlic, rosemary and spices, and top with the remaining scallions and cabbage. Drizzle with water and tamari.
2. In a large pan, add 1-inch of water and boil. Set the steamer basket in the pan of boiling water.

3. Cover and steam for 15 to 20 minutes.

Steamed Mahi Mahi

This entire meal, which is prepared in a simple and quick manner, makes an elegant supper or dinner.

MAKES: 2 servings
PREPARATION TIME: 15 minutes
COOKING TIME: 5 minutes

---

2 bunches Fresh Asparagus, trimmed
2 (4-ounce) Mahi Mahi Fillets
4-6 Scallions, sliced thinly
2 small Carrots, peeled and shredded
2 Garlic Cloves, minced
1 teaspoon Fresh Ginger, minced
1 tablespoon Fresh Lemon juice
1 tablespoon Apple Cider Vinegar
¼ teaspoon Chili powder
Sea Salt, to taste
Freshly Ground Black Pepper, to taste

Directions:

1. Arrange a large sheet of baking paper on a smooth surface and place the fish fillets on the baking paper. Top with the vegetables, except for the asparagus, and drizzle with the lemon juice and vinegar. Sprinkle with the spices. Fold the baking paper to seal the packet around fish and vegetables.
2. Place the asparagus into a bamboo steamer basket and

arrange the fish packet over the asparagus.

3. In a large pan, add 1-inch of water and bring to the boil. Set the steamer basket into the pan of boiling water and steam, covered, for 4 to 5 minutes.

Grilled Tangy Tuna

This recipe makes a simple and tasty tuna grilled dish. The citrus and fresh herb flavors combine nicely with the subtle smokiness from the grilling.

MAKES: 4 servings
PREPARATION TIME: 15 minutes (plus time to marinate)
COOKING TIME: 16 minutes

---

1 tablespoon Fresh Lemon juice
1 tablespoon Fresh Lime juice
2 tablespoons Olive Oil
2 Garlic Cloves, minced
1 tablespoon Fresh Thyme, chopped
1 tablespoon Fresh Basil, chopped
Sea Salt, to taste
Freshly Ground Black Pepper, to taste
4 (4-ounce) Tuna Steaks

Directions:

1. In a bowl, mix together all of the ingredients, except for the tuna. Add the tuna and generously coat with the marinade. Cover the bowl and let the tuna marinate in the refrigerator for at least 1 hour.
2. Preheat the grill to a medium-high heat, and grease the grill grate.
3. Cook for 6 to 8 minutes on both sides.

Mahi Mahi in Parsley Sauce

Mahi Mahi is one of the best fishes for grilling. The parsley sauce made with this recipe wonderfully enhances the flavor of this delicious dish.

MAKES: 4 servings
PREPARATION TIME: 20 minutes (plus time to marinate)
COOKING TIME: 10 minutes

For Fish:
3 Garlic Cloves, chopped
1 Jalapeño Pepper, seeded
½ tablespoon Fresh Oregano, chopped
¼ cup Fresh Lemon Juice
Sea Salt, to taste
Freshly Ground Black Pepper, to taste
4 (6-ounce) Mahi Mahi Fillets

For Tangy Sauce:
½ cup Fresh Parsley Leaves
1 Shallot, sliced
1 Garlic Clove, chopped
1 tablespoon Capers
½ Jalapeño Pepper, seeded
3 tablespoons Fresh Lemon Juice
2 teaspoons Apple Cider Vinegar
3 tablespoons Olive Oil
2 tablespoons Water
Sea Salt, to taste
Freshly Ground Black Pepper, to taste

Directions:

1. Place all of the fish ingredients, except for the fish, into a blender and pulse until smooth. Place the smooth mixture into a large bowl. Add the fish fillets and generously coat with the marinade. Cover and refrigerate to marinate for 30 to 40 minutes.
2. Preheat the grill to a medium heat and grease the grill grate. Remove the fillets from the marinade and shake off any access marinade. Place the fillets on a grill. Cover and cook for 3 to 5 minutes per side.
3. Meanwhile, in a food processor, bland together all of the sauce ingredients until smooth. Place the grilled fish fillets onto a serving plate and serve alongside the sauce.

Lemony Snapper Peak

This is a super healthy and great tasting fish with the touch of lemon and rosemary. Grilling the fish in this recipe ensures you have a moist fish to enjoy.

MAKES: 2 servings
PREPARATION TIME: 10 minutes
COOKING TIME: 15 minutes

4 (5-ounce) Snapper Fillets
Sea Salt, to taste
Freshly Ground Black Pepper, to taste
4 teaspoons Olive Oil
2 tablespoons Fresh Lemon Juice
4 Lemon Slices
4 Sprigs Fresh Rosemary

Directions:

1. Preheat the grill to a medium heat.
2. Place the snapper fillets over 4 heavy-duty aluminum foil sheets. Drizzle the fish with the oil and lemon juice. Arrange the lemon slices and the rosemary sprigs over the snapper fillets, and season with salt and pepper.
3. Fold the foil to seal the packet around fish and grill for 12 to 15 minutes.

Grilled Tilapia Parcel

Grilling fish with vegetables in a foil parcel is a foolproof way to get moist, tender and delicious fish. The tilapia in this recipe combines nicely with the vegetables.

MAKES: 4 servings
PREPARATION TIME: 15 minutes
COOKING TIME: 8 minutes

1 cup Fresh Green Beans, trimmed and cut into 1-inch pieces
1 cup Zucchini, diced
1 cup Cherry Tomatoes, quartered
1 cup Red Onion, sliced thinly
2 teaspoons Capers
2 tablespoons Fresh Parsley, chopped
2 tablespoons Fresh Lime juice
1 tablespoon Olive Oil
Sea Salt, to taste
Freshly Ground Black Pepper, to taste
4 (4-ounce) Tilapia Fillets

Directions:

1. Preheat the grill to a medium heat and grease 4 heavy-duty foil sheets.
2. In a large bowl, except for the fish, mix together all of the ingredients.
3. Arrange the fillets over the prepared foil paper and sprinkle with salt and black pepper. Spoon the vegetable mixture evenly over the fillets. Fold the foil to seal the packet around fish and vegetables and grill for 5 to 8

minutes.

Grilled Scallops

This is a simple, quick, and a very tasty dish. These grilled scallops will have a fantastic smoky flavor.

MAKES: 4 servings
PREPARATION TIME: 15 minutes (plus time to marinate)
COOKING TIME: 6 minutes

1 tablespoon Fresh Lemon juice
1 tablespoon Apple Cider Vinegar
½ tablespoon Fresh Ginger, minced
Sea Salt, to taste
Freshly Ground Black Pepper, to taste
1 pound large Sea Scallops

Directions:

1. In a bowl, mix together all of the ingredients. Cover and refrigerate to marinate for at least 30 to 40 minutes.
2. Preheat the grill to a medium heat and grease the grill grate.
3. Remove the scallops from the marinade, and shake off any access marinade. Place the scallops under the grill, cover, and cook for 2 to 3 minutes per side.

Grilled Salmon Vegetable Kebabs

Grilled Salmon is a delicious and health way to eat fish. This dish will be a great addition to a barbecue party or whenever you wish.

MAKES: 4 servings
PREPARATION TIME: 15 minutes (plus time to marinate)
COOKING TIME: 10 minutes

For the Fish:
1 teaspoon finely diced Fresh Ginger
4-5 Garlic Cloves, minced
2 tablespoons minced Fresh Thyme
½ tablespoon Lime Zest, freshly grated
½ tablespoon Lemon Zest, freshly grated
3 tablespoons Tamari
2 tablespoons Olive Oil
1 tablespoon Fresh Lime juice
1 tablespoon Fresh Lemon juice
Sea Salt, to taste
Freshly Ground Black Pepper, to taste
1½ pounds Salmon Fillets, cubed into 1-inch pieces

For the Vegetables
1 Red Onion, cut into 1-inch pieces
1 Green Bell Pepper, seeded and cut into 1-inch pieces
1 Red Bell Pepper, seeded and cut into 1-inch pieces
Sea Salt, to taste
Freshly Ground Black Pepper, to taste

Directions:

1. In a large bowl, mix together all of the marinade ingredients, except for the fish. Add the salmon and generously coat with the marinade. Place the salmon dish, covered, into the refrigerator to marinate for at least 30 minutes.
2. Preheat the grill to a medium-high heat and grease the grill grate.
3. In a bowl, add the bell peppers and onion, and sprinkle with salt and black pepper. Remove the fish from refrigerator. Discard any excess marinade. Thread the fish, bell pepper and onion pieces onto the pre-soaked wooden skewers.
4. Cook for 4 to 5 minutes on either side, or until the salmon is fully cooked.

Grilled Shrimp with Bulgur

This recipe will make a fresh and healthy combination of bulgur and shrimp with hints of basil and lemon. Your whole family may enjoy this dish.

MAKES: 4 servings
PREPARATION TIME: 20 minutes (plus time to soak)
COOKING TIME: 4 minutes

For the Bulgur:
1½ cups Boiling Water
½ cup Bulgur
2 scallions, chopped
¾ cup Baby Spinach
2 tablespoons diced Fresh Basil Leaves
1 Garlic Clove, minced
¼ cup Olive Oil
¼ cup Fresh Lemon juice
Sea Salt, to taste
Freshly Ground Black Pepper, to taste

For Shrimp:
¼ cup Olive Oil
¼ cup Fresh Lemon juice
2 tablespoons diced Fresh Basil Leaves
Sea Salt, to taste
Freshly Ground Black Pepper, to taste
1 pound large Shrimp, peeled and deveined

Directions:

1. In a large bowl, combine the boiling water with the bulgur. Cover and set aside for 1 to 2 hours. Drain the excess water. Add the scallions, spinach, basil and garlic. Drizzle with oil and lemon juice, and season with black pepper and salt.
2. Mix together all of the shrimp ingredients in a bowl. Set aside for 10 to 15 minutes.
3. Preheat the grill to a high heat and grease the grill grate. Cook the shrimp for 1 to 2 minutes on either side.
4. On a serving plate, place the bulgur mixture and top with the shrimp before serving.

POULTRY RECIPES

Roasted Chicken Squash

This baked chicken and butternut squash is a delicious dish. The vinegar sauce provides the perfect counterpart to the chicken.

MAKES: 4 servings
PREPARATION TIME: 15 minutes
COOKING TIME: 30 minutes

4 (4-ounce) skinless, boneless Chicken Breasts
Sea Salt, to taste
Freshly Ground Black Pepper, to taste
1½ pounds peeled, seeded and cubed Summer Squash
1 tablespoon Fresh Thyme, chopped
1 tablespoon Fresh Rosemary, chopped
2 teaspoons Apple Cider Vinegar

For Sauce:
1 Garlic Clove, minced
2 teaspoons Fresh Ginger, minced
2 teaspoons Apple Cider Vinegar

Directions:

1. Preheat the oven to 400 degrees F. Arrange the rack on the lower third of the oven. Line a roasting pan with parchment paper.
2. Place the chicken breasts onto the prepared pan and generously sprinkle with salt and black pepper. Arrange the squash cubes around the chicken, and sprinkle the squash with salt and black pepper. Top with chopped herbs and drizzle with the vinegar. Roast for about 15 minutes.
3. Meanwhile, in a bowl, mix together all of the sauce ingredients. Flip the chicken and coat generously with the sauce. Flip the squash and bake for a further 15 minutes.

Chicken & White Bean Stew

This recipe makes a delicious and hearty meal. Enjoy this protein-rich dish that is filled with the delicious flavors of chicken, white beans and herbs.

MAKES: 4 servings
PREPARATION TIME: 15 minutes
COOKING TIME: 25 minutes

---

3 cups Homemade Chicken Broth
1 medium Onion, chopped
1 Garlic Clove, minced
4 (4-ounce) skinless, boneless Chicken Breasts
1½ cups Cooked White Beans
1 teaspoon Dried Thyme, crushed
1 teaspoon Dried Oregano, crushed
1 teaspoon Cayenne Pepper
Sea Salt, to taste
Freshly Ground Black Pepper, to taste
2 tablespoons Fresh Parsley, chopped

Directions:

1. In a large soup pan, heat 2 tablespoons of broth on a medium heat. Add the garlic and onion and boil for 4 to 5 minutes.
2. Add the chicken and return to the boil. Once boiling reduce the heat and simmer for 15 minutes, covered, or until the chicken has become tender. Transfer the

chicken onto a plate and cut the chicken into bite size pieces.

3. Add the remaining ingredients and chicken pieces to the pan. Return to the boil on a medium heat. Reduce the heat, cover and simmer for a further 5 minutes.

Tomato Baked Chicken

This is a hit recipe for a delicious meal. The fresh herbs provide a wonderful taste to complement the chicken and cherry tomatoes.

MAKES: 4 servings
PREPARATION TIME: 15 minutes
COOKING TIME: 55 minutes

---

4 (4-ounce) skinless, boneless Chicken Breasts
2 cups Grape Tomatoes
2 tablespoons Fresh Oregano, chopped
2 tablespoons Fresh Rosemary, chopped
1 tablespoon Fresh Lime juice
1 tablespoon Olive Oil
Sea Salt, to taste
Freshly Ground Black Pepper, to taste

Directions:

1. Preheat the oven to 425 degrees F and line a large baking dish with parchment paper.
2. Place the chicken breasts onto the prepared baking dish in a single layer. Place the tomatoes and herbs over the chicken. Drizzle with lime juice and oil, and sprinkle with salt and black pepper.
3. Bake for 45 to 55 minutes.

Curried Coconut Chicken

This is an easy and exotic chicken breast recipe. The ground turmeric gives the chicken a beautiful color in this dish.

MAKES: 2 servings
PREPARATION TIME: 15 minutes
COOKING TIME: 1 hour

2 (4-ounce) skinless, boneless Chicken Breast halves
1 small Red Bell Pepper, seeded and diced
1 small Green Bell Pepper, seeded and diced
½ White Onion, diced
2 tablespoons Coconut Oil, melted
¼ teaspoon Ground Turmeric
¼ teaspoon Cayenne Pepper
Sea Salt, to taste
Freshly Ground Black Pepper, to taste

Directions:

1. Preheat the oven to 350 degrees F and line a small baking dish with foil.
2. Arrange the chicken breast halves in the prepared baking dish. Spread the bell peppers and onion over the chicken. Sprinkle with the spices and drizzle with oil.
3. Cover the baking dish with foil and bake for 45 to 60 minutes.

Crispy Chicken

Baking the chicken gives this dish a moist and beautifully golden coating, as well as a deliciously crunchy texture. This is an easy recipe for a great weeknight meal.

MAKES: 2 servings
PREPARATION TIME: 15 minutes
COOKING TIME: 25 minute

4 Egg Whites, beaten
1 teaspoon Dried Rosemary, crushed
¼ teaspoon Cayenne Pepper
Sea Salt, to taste
Freshly Ground Black Pepper, to taste
½ cup Coconut Flour
2 (4-ounce) skinless, boneless Chicken Breasts

Directions:

1. Preheat the oven to 400 degrees F and grease a baking dish.
2. In a shallow dish, beat together the egg whites, rosemary, cayenne, salt and black pepper. In another shallow dish, place the coconut flour. Dip the chicken breasts in the egg mixture before rolling in the coconut flour.
3. Place the breasts onto the prepared baking dish and bake for 20 to 25 minutes.

Stuffed Chicken Breasts

This recipe presents a new way to prepare a healthy and delicious chicken dish. This easy recipe makes chicken breasts more desirable.

MAKES: 4 servings
PREPARATION TIME: 15 minutes
COOKING TIME: 20 minutes

¼ cup tomatoes, seeded and finely chopped
2 Garlic Cloves, minced
2 teaspoons Lime Zest, freshly grated
1 tablespoon Mixed Dried Herbs (rosemary, thyme, oregano), crushed
Sea Salt, to taste
Freshly Ground Black Pepper, to taste
2 tablespoons Olive Oil
4 skinless, boneless Chicken Breast Halves
2 tablespoons Fresh Lime juice

Directions:

1. Preheat the grill to a medium heat and grease the grill grate.
2. In a large bowl, mix together the tomatoes, garlic, lime zest, herbs, salt and black pepper. With a sharp knife, cut horizontally through half of the chicken breasts to form a slit. Evenly fill each chicken breast with the tomato mixture. Drizzle the beasts with lime juice, and sprinkle with a little salt and black pepper.
3. Arrange the chicken breasts on the grill grate and grill

for 10 minutes each side.

Tangy Chicken Tenders

Lemon gives a refreshingly tangy touch to these chicken tenders.
The use of cilantro in the sauce also beautifully enhances the
flavor of the grilled chicken.

MAKES: 4 servings
PREPARATION TIME: 20 minutes (plus time to marinate)
COOKING TIME: 8 minutes

For Chicken:
1 tablespoon Olive Oil
2 tablespoons Fresh Lemon juice
2 teaspoons Lemon Zest, freshly grated
Sea Salt, to taste
Freshly Ground Black Pepper, to taste
1 pound skinless, boneless Chicken Breast Tenders

For Tangy Sauce:
2 tablespoon Fresh Lemon juice
1 tablespoon Apple Cider Vinegar
2 tablespoons Olive Oil
1 tablespoon Onion, chopped
½ cup Fresh Cilantro, chopped
Sea Salt, to taste
Freshly Ground Black Pepper, to taste

Directions:

1. For the chicken, in a bowl mix together all of the ingredients, except for the chicken. Add the chicken and generously coat with the marinade. Cover and set aside for at least 20 to 25 minutes.
2. Preheat the grill to a medium heat and grease the grill grate. Shake off any excess marinade from the chicken, and place the chicken onto the grill. Grill for about 8 minutes, flipping once after 4 minutes.
3. Meanwhile, in a blender, add all of the sauce ingredients and pulse until smooth. Serve the chicken tenders alongside the sauce.

Grilled Citrus Chicken

The use of lemon and lime juice with herbs in this recipe adds a refreshingly delicious citrus flavor to the chicken.

MAKES: 4 servings
PREPARATION TIME: 15 minutes (plus time to marinate)
COOKING TIME: 20 minutes

---

2 tablespoons Olive Oil
2 tablespoons Fresh Lime juice
2 tablespoons Fresh Lemon juice
1 teaspoon Fresh Lime Zest, freshly grated
1 teaspoon Fresh Lemon Zest, freshly grated
1 teaspoon Garlic, minced
½ teaspoon Dried Oregano, crushed
1 teaspoon Dried Thyme, crushed
Sea Salt, to taste
Freshly Ground Black Pepper, to taste
4 skinless, boneless Chicken Breasts

Directions:

1. In a large mixing bowl, mix together all of the ingredients, except the chicken breasts. Add the chicken and generously coat with the marinade. Cover and refrigerate for 8 to 10 hours.
2. Grill the chicken under a medium-high heat for 9 to 10 minutes each side.

Broiled Chicken with Carrots

This is a simple but delicious way to prepare a tasty and healthy chicken. The combination of herbs and lemon adds wonderful flavors to the chicken.

MAKES: 2 servings
PREPARATION TIME: 15 minutes (plus time to marinate)
COOKING TIME: 17 minutes

2 Garlic Cloves, minced
1 teaspoon Lemon Zest, freshly grated
½ tablespoon Fresh Sage, chopped
½ tablespoon Fresh Oregano, chopped
2 (4-ounce) skinless, boneless Chicken Breast Halves
3 Carrots, peeled and cut into 1-inch pieces
1 tablespoon Olive Oil
Sea Salt, to taste
Freshly Ground Black Pepper, to taste

Directions:

1. In a large bowl, mix together the garlic, lemon zest and herbs. Add the chicken and rub with the herb mixture. Set aside for 15 to 20 minutes.
2. Preheat the grill and set the rack 6-inches away from the heating element. Line a baking pan with foil.
3. Place the chicken breasts onto the prepared baking pan. Arrange carrot pieces around the chicken and drizzle the chicken and carrots with oil. Sprinkle with salt and black pepper.

4. Grill for about 7 minutes. Flip the chicken and grill for a further 8 to 10 minutes.

Chicken & Onion Kebabs

These tangy flavored chicken and onion kebabs are a perfect hit for the long weekends. The delicious kick of these kebabs comes from the lemon and herbs.

MAKES: 4 servings
PREPARATION TIME: 15 minutes (plus time to marinate)
COOKING TIME: 10 minutes

¼ cup Olive Oil
3 tablespoons Fresh Lemon juice
4 Garlic Cloves, minced
2 teaspoons Lemon Zest, freshly grated
1 teaspoon Dried Oregano, crushed
1 teaspoon Dried Thyme, crushed
¼ teaspoon Cayenne Pepper
Sea Salt, to taste
Freshly Ground Black Pepper, to taste
1½ pounds skinless, boneless cubed Chicken Breast Halves
1 large Green Bell Pepper, seeded and cut into 1-inch cubes
1 Red Onion, cut into 1-inch cubes

Directions:

1. In a large bowl, mix together 2 tablespoons of oil, 1 tablespoon of lemon juice, garlic, lemon zest, herbs and spices. Add the chicken and generously coat with the oil mixture. Cover and set aside for 30 to 40 minutes. In another small bowl, mix together the remaining oil and

lemon juice.
2. Preheat the barbecue to a medium-high heat. Take the chicken pieces from the marinade and discard any excess marinade. Thread the chicken, bell pepper and onion pieces onto metal skewers.
3. Cook for about 9 to 10 minutes, turning and occasionally coating the kebabs with the lemon mixture.

Creamy Chicken Strips

These marinated chicken skewers are a great hit for any gathering. The marinade compliments the tender chicken very nicely.

MAKES: 4 servings
PREPARATION TIME: 15 minutes (plus time to marinate)
COOKING TIME: 8 minutes

For Chicken

1 large Onion, chopped
3-4 Garlic Cloves, chopped
2 tablespoons Fresh Ginger, chopped
1 Serrano Pepper, stemmed and chopped
¼ teaspoon Cayenne Pepper
Sea salt, to taste
Freshly Ground Black Pepper, to taste
¼ cup Coconut Oil, melted
4-ounces skinless, boneless, strips of Chicken Breast

For Sauce

1½ cups Almond Milk, unsweetened
¼ cup Natural Peanut Butter
2 tablespoons Homemade Chicken Broth
2 tablespoons Fresh Lemon juice

Directions:

1. In a food processor, add all of the chicken ingredients, except for the chicken, and pulse until a smooth paste forms. Transfer half of the mixture into a large bowl, reserving the other half. Add the chicken strips and coat with the marinade. Cover and refrigerate to marinate for about 1 hour.
2. Preheat the grill to a medium heat and grease the grill grate. Thread the chicken strips onto skewers. Grill the chicken strips for about 3 to 4 minutes each side.
3. Meanwhile, in a pan, add the reserved onion mixture and heat on a medium heat. Cook, stirring, for 3 to 4 minutes before stirring in all of the sauce ingredients. Reduce the heat and cook, stirring, for a further 3 to 4 minutes, or until the sauce is thick and creamy.
4. To serve, place the chicken skewers on a serving plate and top with the sauce.

Marinated Chicken Gala

This steamed chicken recipe will make a moist, delicious and healthy meal. The cabbage in this recipe adds extra juices to give the dish a unique taste.

MAKES: 4 servings
PREPARATION TIME: 15 minutes (plus time to marinate)
COOKING TIME: 15 minutes

1 cup Fresh Parsley Leaves, chopped
1 Garlic Clove, minced
½ teaspoon Fresh Ginger, minced
1 cup Tamari
1 tablespoon Fresh Lemon juice
2 tablespoons Olive Oil
Sea salt, to taste
Freshly Ground Black Pepper, to taste
4 (4-ounce) boneless, skinless Chicken Breasts
1 Head Cabbage leaves separated

Directions:

1. In a large bowl, mix together all of the ingredients, except the chicken and cabbage. Add the chicken and generously coat with the marinade before covering and refrigerating overnight.
2. In a large pan, add 1-inch of water and boil. Place the cabbage leaves into the bottom of a bamboo steamer. Arrange the chicken breasts over the cabbage leaves and

set the steamer into the pan of boiling water.
3. Cover and steam for 10 to 15 minutes.

Chicken Vegetable Wraps

These salad wraps are tantalizingly delicious. They are also really light and full of fresh vegetable flavors.

MAKES: 2 servings
PREPARATION TIME: 20 minutes

1 cup Grilled Chicken, chopped
½ cup Green Bell Pepper, seeded and sliced thinly
¼ cup Tomatoes, seeded and sliced thinly
¼ cup Red Onion, sliced thinly
2 tablespoons finely diced Fresh Cilantro Leaves
1 teaspoon Apple Cider Vinegar
Sea salt, to taste
Freshly Ground Black Pepper, to taste
2 large Fresh Iceberg Lettuce Leaves

Directions:

1. In a large bowl, except for the lettuce, mix together all of the ingredients.
2. Spoon the chicken and vegetable mixture evenly into the lettuce leaves.
3. Roll the leaves and serve.

Baked Turkey Patties

This is a simply fabulous and delicious recipe for turkey patties.
These patties are loaded with rich flavors.

MAKES: 4 servings
PREPARATION TIME: 10 minutes
COOKING TIME: 30 minutes

1 pound Lean Ground Turkey
1 Egg White
1 Garlic Clove, minced
1 Scallion, finely chopped
3 tablespoons diced Parsley Leaves
¼ teaspoon Chilli Powder
Sea Salt, to taste
Freshly Ground Black Pepper, to taste

Directions:

1. Preheat the oven to 350 degrees F and line a cookie sheet with parchment paper.
2. In a large bowl, mix together all of the ingredients. Make your desired size patties from the turkey mixture. Place the patties onto the prepared cookie sheet in a single layer.
3. Bake for about 30 minutes.

Baked Turkey Meatballs

Baked turkey meatballs are a neat and tidy way to use lean turkey. These meatballs are positively mouthwatering.

MAKES: 4 servings
PREPARATION TIME: 15 minutes
COOKING TIME: 20 minutes

1 pound Lean Ground Turkey
½ cup Carrot, peeled and finely grated
1 Garlic Clove, minced
2 tablespoons diced Cilantro Leaves
1 large Egg White, beaten
2 tablespoons Almond Flour
Sea Salt, to taste
Freshly Ground Black Pepper, to taste

Directions:

1. Preheat the oven to 350 degrees F and line a baking sheet with parchment paper.
2. In a large bowl, mix together all of the ingredients. Make your desired size balls from the turkey mixture. Arrange balls on the prepared baking sheet in a single layer.
3. Bake for 15 to 20 minutes.

MEAT RECIPES

Hearty Beef Stew

This is a warming, hearty and a wonderfully flavorful stew. The meat is cooked in a pressure cooker with vegetables and herbs in a hearty broth.

MAKES: 4 servings
PREPARATION TIME: 20 minutes
COOKING TIME: 50 minutes

---

4 cups Beef Broth
1 pound Beef Stew Meat, trimmed and cubed
1 teaspoon Dried Thyme, crushed
1 teaspoon Dried Oregano, crushed
½ teaspoon Cayenne Pepper
Sea Salt, to taste
Freshly Ground Black Pepper, to taste
1 Onion, chopped
2 Celery Stalks, chopped
1 tablespoon Garlic, chopped
2 tablespoons Olive Oil
2 teaspoons Fresh Rosemary, chopped
3 Turnips, peeled and cubed
3 Parsnips, peeled and cubed
2 cups Kale, trimmed and chopped

¼ cup Fresh Cilantro, chopped

Directions:

1. In a pressure cooker, heat ¼ cup of the broth on a medium-high heat. Add the meat and cook for 4 to 5 minutes. Transfer the meat onto a plate. Add the onion, celery and garlic into the pressure cooker and cook for 4 to 5 minutes.
2. Return the beef to the pot and then add the remaining broth, oil and all seasonings. Cover and cook for about 20 minutes, reducing the heat to medium-low after a steady stream of steam is emitted from the valve of the pressure cooker.
3. Uncover and stir in the turnips, parsnips and kale. Cover and cook for 20 minutes more. Top with parsley and serve hot.

Spicy Grilled Flank

This is a simple yet delicious dinner idea. The combination of using a spice marinade and grilling the meat works really well on this flank steak.

MAKES: 4 servings
PREPARATION TIME: 10 minutes (plus time to marinate)
COOKING TIME: 10 minutes

¼ teaspoon Cayenne Pepper
Sea Salt, to taste
Freshly Ground Black Pepper, to taste
1 (1-pound) Flank Steak, trimmed

Directions:

1. In a large bowl, mix together the cayenne pepper, salt and black pepper. Generously rub the spice mixture over the steak. Cover and set aside to marinate for 15 to 20 minutes.
2. Preheat the grill and place the rack 4-inches from heat element. Grease the grill pan.
3. Place the steak on the prepared grill pan and grill for 4 to 5 minutes per side.

Tangy Grill Delight

This recipe makes one of the best and most delicious mid-week meals for the whole family. Fresh lime adds a great taste to this steak.

MAKES: 4 servings
PREPARATION TIME: 10 minutes
COOKING TIME: 15 minutes

1 tablespoon Fresh Lime juice
2 Garlic Cloves, minced
½ teaspoon Lime Zest, freshly grated
1 teaspoon Fresh Rosemary, chopped
Sea Salt, to taste
Freshly Ground Black Pepper, to taste
2 (4-ounce) Sirloin Steaks

Directions:

1. Preheat the grill and place the rack 4-inches from heat element. Grease the grill pan.
2. In a large bowl, add the garlic, lime juice, lime zest and spices. Add the steaks and generously coat with the garlic mixture.
3. Grill the steaks for 14 to 15 minutes, turning once after about 7 minutes.

Grilled Herb Steak

This is a great way to prepare flank steak. The fresh, tangy and herbed marinade infuses a wonderful flavor in the beef.

MAKES: 4 servings
PREPARATION TIME: 15 minutes (plus time to marinate)
COOKING TIME: 14 minutes

---

1 tablespoon Fresh Lemon juice
1 tablespoon Fresh Lime juice
2 tablespoons Olive Oil
¼ cup White Onion, minced
1 Garlic Clove, minced
1 teaspoon Lemon Zest, freshly grated
¼ teaspoon Dried Basil, crushed
⅛ teaspoon Dried Oregano, crushed
⅛ teaspoon Dried Thyme, crushed
Sea Salt, to taste
Freshly Ground Black Pepper, to taste
½ pound Flank Steak

Directions:

1. In a large bowl, mix together all of the ingredients, except for the steak. Add the steak and generously coat with the marinade. Cover and refrigerate to marinate for 8 to 10 hours, tossing occasionally. Remove from the refrigerator and sit at room temperature for 15 to 20 minutes.

2. Preheat the grill to a medium heat and grease the grill grate.
3. Remove any excess marinade from the steaks, and place them under the grill. Grill for about 7 minutes on either side.

Chili Grilled Steak

This is a perfect and delicious addition to your menu repertoire. The simple blend of spices makes for a wonderfully tasty flank steak.

MAKES: 4 servings
PREPARATION TIME: 15 minutes (plus time to marinate)
COOKING TIME: 8 minutes

½ teaspoon Ground Cinnamon
1 teaspoon Chipotle Chile Powder
1 teaspoon Chili Powder
Sea Salt, to taste
Freshly Ground Black Pepper, to taste
2 pounds Flank Iron Steak, trimmed

Directions:

1. In a large bowl, mix together all of the spices. Add the steak and generously rub with the spice mixture. Cover and refrigerate to marinate for at least 6 to 8 hours.
2. Preheat the grill to a medium-high heat, and grease the grill grate.
3. Place the steaks under the grill and cook for about 4 minutes each side.

Gingery Short Ribs

This recipe is perfect for quickly making tasty grilled short ribs.
Enjoy this quick dinner whenever you're pressed for time and still
want a healthy dinner.

MAKES: 4 servings
PREPARATION TIME: 10 minutes (plus time to marinate)
COOKING TIME: 8 minutes

3 tablespoons Fresh Ginger, finely grated
5-6 Garlic Cloves, minced
½ cup Tamari
1 tablespoon Fresh Lemon juice
Sea Salt, to taste
Freshly Ground Black Pepper, to taste
2 pounds boneless Short Ribs, trimmed

Directions:

1. In a large bowl, mix together all of the ingredients, except for the ribs. Add the ribs and generously coat with the marinade. Cover and refrigerate to marinate for at least 4 to 5 hours.
2. Preheat the grill to a high heat and grease the grill grate.
3. Place the ribs under the grill and cook for 3 to 4 minutes either side.

Savory Roasted Beef

This delicious marinade is a combination of sweet, savory and tangy ingredients. It adds a fantastic flavoring into these short ribs.

MAKES: 4 servings
PREPARATION TIME: 15 minutes (plus time to marinate)
COOKING TIME: 2 hours

½ cup Tamari
½ cup Unsweetened Applesauce
2 tablespoon Apple Cider vinegar
2 tablespoons Fresh Lime juice
½ cup Homemade Beef Broth
2 Scallions, chopped
2 tablespoons Garlic, minced
2 tablespoons Fresh Ginger, minced
Sea Salt, to taste
Freshly Ground Black Pepper, to taste
4 pounds Beef Short Ribs, trimmed

Directions:

1. In a large bowl, mix together all of the ingredients, except for the ribs. Add the ribs and generously coat with the marinade. Cover the bowl and refrigerate for at least 24 hours.
2. Preheat the oven to 300 degrees F. Transfer the ribs with marinade in a Dutch oven.

3. Roast for about 2 hours, or until cooked.

Herb Roasted Sirloin

This is a simple and easy recipe for roast sirloin. The combination
of the marinade with the sirloin gives a lovely rich flavor.

MAKES: 4 servings
PREPARATION TIME: 15 minutes (plus time to marinate)
COOKING TIME: 1 hour

2 tablespoons Fresh Lime juice
1 tablespoon Olive Oil
2 Garlic Cloves, minced
1 tablespoon Fresh Rosemary, chopped
1 tablespoon Fresh Basil, chopped
¼ teaspoon Chili Powder
Sea Salt, to taste
Freshly Ground Black Pepper, to taste
2 pounds Sirloin Tip Roast, trimmed

Directions:

1. In a large bowl, mix together all of the ingredients, except for the sirloin. Add the sirloin and generously coat with the marinade. Cover and set aside for at least 30 to 40 minutes.
2. Preheat the oven to 325 degrees F and place the rack on the upper part of the oven. Place the sirloin into the roasting pan and cook for 50 to 60 minutes.

Kebabs Haven

This is another clean and healthy beef recipe which also happens to make a quick meal. This recipe will create delicious, aromatic and spicy beef kebabs.

MAKES: 4 servings
PREPARATION TIME: 15 minutes (plus time to marinate)
COOKING TIME: 15 minutes

---

3 Garlic Cloves, minced
1 tablespoon Fresh Parsley, minced
2 tablespoons Homemade Beef Broth
1 teaspoon Chili Powder
Sea Salt, to taste
Freshly Ground Black Pepper, to taste
1½ pounds Beef Sirloin, trimmed and cubed into ½-inch size
3 tablespoons Olive Oil

Directions:

1. In a large bowl, mix together all of the ingredients, except for the beef and oil. Add the beef and generously coat with marinade. Cover and refrigerate to marinate for at least 2 to 3 hours.
2. Preheat the grill to a high heat and grease the grill grate.
3. Thread the beef onto pre-soaked wooden skewers. Place the oil in a plate and coat the skewers with the oil evenly. Place the skewers under the grill. Cook the kebabs for 12 to 15 minutes and turn occasionally.

E-Zee Lamb Chops

This recipe will help you make quick and delicious lamb chops.

MAKES: 2 servings
PREPARATION TIME: 10 minutes
COOKING TIME: 8 minutes

4 (4-ounce) Lamb Loin Chops, trimmed
Sea salt, to taste
Freshly Ground Black Pepper, to taste

Directions:

1. Preheat the grill to a medium-high heat and lightly grease the grill grate.
2. Generously rub the chops with the salt and black pepper.
3. Grill the chops for 3 to 4 minutes either side.

Crispy Baked Lamb Chops

This recipe is a great and is worth every minute of your time. It is an easy way to make crispy chops which are very tasty, yet with just a few ingredients.

MAKES: 4 servings
PREPARATION TIME: 15 minutes
COOKING TIME: 40 minutes

5 Egg Whites
Sea Salt, to taste
Freshly Ground Black Pepper, to taste
2 cups Whole Wheat Breadcrumbs
8 Lamb Chops, trimmed

Directions:

1. Preheat the oven to 375 degrees F and grease a baking dish.
2. In a shallow dish, mix together the egg whites, salt and black pepper. Place the breadcrumbs into a separate shallow dish. Dip the chops into the egg white mixture and then roll them in the breadcrumbs.
3. Place the chops into the prepared baking dish and bake for about 40 minutes, turn the chops after 20 minutes.

Sour Spice Grilled Lamb

The combination of vinegar and herbs balances the richness of these spicy grilled chops. This recipe will make a nice dish for the whole family.

MAKES: 4 servings
PREPARATION TIME: 15 minutes (plus time to marinate)
COOKING TIME: 10 minutes

2 Garlic Cloves, minced
1 tablespoon Fresh Thyme, chopped
1 tablespoon Fresh Oregano, chopped
¼ cup Apple Cider Vinegar
2 tablespoons Olive Oil
Sea Salt, to taste
Freshly Ground Black Pepper, to taste
8 Lamb Rib Chops, trimmed

Directions:

1. In a large bowl, mix together all of the ingredients, except for the chops. Add the chops and generously coat with the marinade. Cover and refrigerate for at least 1 to 2 hours.
2. Preheat the grill to a medium-high heat and grease the grill grate.
3. Grill the chops for 5 minutes either side.

Zesty Lamb Chops

The combination of lemon and lime in this recipe will make these chops so flavorful that maybe even those who don't usually like lamb may come back for more.

MAKES: 4 servings
PREPARATION TIME: 15 minutes (plus time to marinate)
COOKING TIME: 8 minutes

1 tablespoon Fresh Lime juice
1 tablespoon Fresh Lemon juice
2 tablespoons Olive Oil
2 tablespoons Garlic, minced
½ teaspoon Lime Zest, freshly grated
½ teaspoon Lemon Zest, freshly grated
2 teaspoons Dried Rosemary, crushed
Sea Salt, to taste
Freshly Ground Black Pepper, to taste
8 (4-ounce) Lamb Loin Chops, trimmed

Directions:

1. In a large bowl, mix together all of the ingredients, except for the chops. Add the chops and generously coat with marinade. Cover and refrigerate to marinate for at least 1 to 2 hours.
2. Preheat the grill to a medium-high heat and grease the grill grate.
3. Grill the chops for 3 to 4 minutes on either side.

Quick Lamb Deal

This simple spicy marinade gives this dish an intense flavor. These grilled chops may certainly please the entire family.

MAKES: 4 servings
PREPARATION TIME: 15 minutes (plus time to marinate)
COOKING TIME: 8 minutes

3 Garlic cloves, crushed
1 tablespoon diced Fresh Thyme Leaves
½ teaspoon Cayenne Pepper
Pinch of Ground Cinnamon
Sea Salt, to taste
Freshly Ground Black Pepper, to taste
4 Lamb Loin Chops, trimmed

Directions:

1. In a large bowl, mix together all of the ingredients, except for the chops. Add the chops and generously coat with the marinade. Cover and set aside for at least 15 to 20 minutes.
2. Preheat the grill to a medium-high heat and grease the grill grate.
3. Grill the chops for 3 to 4 minutes on either side.

Braise Grilled Lamb

The method of preparing these lamb shanks gives it a beautiful crust with a wonderful flavor. In addition, the sauce made with this dish fantastically enhances the flavor of these shanks.

MAKES: 4 servings
PREPARATION TIME: 15 minutes
COOKING TIME: 2 hours 15 minutes

1 cup Homemade Beef Broth
1 teaspoon Fresh Lemon juice
4 Lamb Shanks, trimmed
6-8 Whole Garlic Cloves, peeled
Sea Salt, to taste
Freshly Ground Black Pepper, to taste

Directions:

1. In a pan, add the broth, lemon juice, the shanks and garlic, and bring to a boil on a high heat. Reduce the heat and simmer, covered, for at least 2 hours, turning the shanks after every 30 minutes. Remove from the heat and transfer the shanks onto a plate. Strain the sauce. Stir in salt and black pepper and reheat the sauce for 2 to 3 minutes.
2. Preheat the grill to a medium-high heat and grease the grill grate.
3. Generously sprinkle the shanks with salt and black pepper. Grill the shanks for 15 minutes and turn occasionally.
4. Serve the shanks with the sauce.

Tangy Marinade Lamb Shanks

These wonderfully delicious lamb shanks are grilled with a coating of a tangy marinade with the combination of tomatoes, garlic, onion and rosemary.

MAKES: 4 servings
PREPARATION TIME: 25 minutes (plus time to marinate)
COOKING TIME: 3 hours 6 minutes

2 cups Homemade Chicken Broth
⅓ cup Olive Oil
¼ cup Fresh Lemon Juice
½ cup Apple Cider Vinegar
2 Plum Tomatoes, chopped
2 Large Onions, chopped
4-5 Garlic Cloves, chopped
1 Bunch Fresh Rosemary, chopped
Sea Salt, to taste
Freshly Ground Black Pepper, to taste
4 Lamb Shanks, trimmed

Directions:

1. In a blender, add all of the ingredients, except for the shanks, and pulse until smooth. Place the marinade mixture into a large bowl. Add the shanks and generously coat with the marinade. Cover and refrigerate for at least 1 to 2 hours.
2. Preheat the grill to a high heat and grease the grill grate.
3. Remove the shanks from the marinade and discard any

excess marinade. Reserve the marinade. Grill the shanks for 2 to 3 minutes either side. Then, place the shanks to the indirect heat. Cover and grill for 2½ to 3 hours, turning and coating the shanks with the reserved marinade every 30 minutes.

Slow Roasted Lamb

This is a great and easy way to enjoy lamb shanks. The slow roasting method makes these shanks incredibly flavorful and succulent.

MAKES: 4 servings
PREPARATION TIME: 15 minutes
COOKING TIME: 2 hours 35 minutes

4 Garlic Cloves, crushed
2 teaspoons Dried Marjoram, crushed
1 tablespoon Fresh Thyme, chopped
1 tablespoon Fresh Oregano, chopped
4 Lamb Shanks, trimmed
2 tablespoons Olive Oil
2 tablespoons Fresh Lime juice
2 tablespoons Fresh Lemon juice
Sea Salt, to taste
Freshly Ground Black Pepper, to taste
1 cup Homemade Chicken Broth

Directions:

1. Preheat the oven to 450 degrees F and grease a large roasting pan.
2. In a bowl, mix together garlic and herbs and set aside. Arrange the shanks in the prepared roasting pan in a single layer. Drizzle with the oil and citrus juices, and sprinkle with the salt and black pepper. Roast the shanks for about 20 minutes.
3. Remove the roasting pan from oven. Reduce the

temperature of oven to 325 degrees F. Sprinkle the shanks with the herb mixture. Cover the roasting pan tightly with aluminum foil and roast for a further 2 hours.

4. Remove the roasting pan from the oven. Increase the temperature of oven to 400 degrees F. Add the chicken broth into the roasting pan and roast for a final 15 minutes.

Lamb Barley Stew

This stew is quick and easy to prepare and is a hearty and warming comfort food. By including barley in this dish it turns out to be an unusual but tasty lamb dish.

MAKES: 4 servings
PREPARATION TIME: 20 minutes
COOKING TIME: 25 minutes

---

6 cups Homemade Chicken Broth
2 pounds Lamb Shanks, trimmed
½ cup Pearl Barley, rinsed and drained
2 Fresh Oregano Sprigs
12 Small Turnips, peeled and cut into bite sized pieces
1 medium Carrot, peeled and cut into bite sized pieces
2 medium Scallions, sliced
½ Head Cabbage, shredded
Sea Salt, to taste
Freshly Ground Black Pepper, to taste

Directions:

1. In a pressure cooker set on a high heat, add the broth, lamb, barley and oregano. Cover and cook for about 20 minutes, reducing the heat to medium after a steady stream of steam is emitted from the valve of the pressure cooker. Remove from the heat, cover, and set aside for 10 minutes.
2. Uncover the cooker and stir in vegetables, salt and black

pepper. Cover and cook for a further 5 minutes. Remove from the heat and set aside, covered, for a further 10 minutes before serving hot.

DESSERT RECIPES

Berries Granita

This soft, light and delicious dessert makes a refreshing after dinner treats. It may be loved by all who taste it!

MAKES: 2 servings
PREPARATION TIME: 10 minutes (plus time to freeze)

½ cup Xylitol or Stevia to taste
½ cup Warm Water
1½ cups Fresh Raspberries
1½ cups Fresh Strawberries, sliced
2 tablespoons Fresh Lemon Juice

Directions:

1. In a blender, add the xylitol and water and pulse until the xylitol has dissolved. Add the berries and the lemon juice, and pulse until smooth. Transfer the mixture into a large bowl. Cover and freeze for at least 3 to 4 hours.
2. Remove from the freezer. With a wooden spoon, stir the dessert until smooth before covering and freezing again.

If possible freeze overnight.

3. Remove from the freezer and set aside at room temperature for at least 10 minutes. With a fork, mix the granita until it becomes creamy and fluffy.

Mini Carrot Cakes

This flavorful carrot cake is moist and loaded with delicious and healthy nutrients. This recipe makes a tasty classic and very easy-to-make cake.

MAKES: 2 servings
PREPARATION TIME: 15 minutes
COOKING TIME: 28 minutes

1⅓ cups Almond Flour
¼ teaspoon Baking Soda
½ teaspoon Ground Cinnamon
Pinch of Sea Salt
2 tablespoons Coconut Oil, melted
⅓ cup Almond Milk, unsweetened
2 large Eggs, Whites only
Liquid Stevia, to taste
1 cup Carrot, peeled and grated

Directions:

1. Preheat the oven to 350 degrees F and grease 2 (12-ounce) ramekins.
2. In a large bowl, mix together the baking soda, flour, cinnamon and salt. In another bowl, add the oil, milk, egg whites and stevia, and beat together. Mix the oil mixture into the flour mixture and fold in the carrot.
3. Transfer the mixture into the prepared ramekins. Bake for 25 to 28 minutes, or until a toothpick inserted into the centre comes out clean.

Raspberry Mousse

This recipe is a delicious way of using fresh raspberries. The use of lemon juice adds subtle flavors into this easy dessert.

MAKES: 2 servings

PREPARATION TIME: 15 minutes (plus time to refrigerate)

¼ cup Cashew nuts, soaked for 2-4 hours and drained
1 pound Fresh Raspberries
¼ cup Coconut Oil, melted
¼ cup Applesauce, unsweetened
2 tablespoons Fresh Lemon juice

Directions:

1. In a blender, add the cashew nuts and pulse until chopped very finely. Add the remaining ingredients and pulse until smooth.
2. Transfer the mixture into serving bowls. Refrigerate to chill completely before serving.

Rhubarb Compote

This rhubarb compote is a great way to use any excess rhubarb in your kitchen. The lemon juice and cinnamon add a wonderful subtle flavor to this quick dessert.

MAKES: 4 servings
PREPARATION TIME: 15 minutes (plus time to refrigerate)
COOKING TIME: 10 minutes

---

3 cups Fresh Rhubarb, cut into small pieces
2 tablespoons Fresh Lemon Juice
¼ teaspoon Ground Cinnamon
Liquid Stevia, to taste
2 Egg Whites

Directions:

1. Add the rhubarb, lemon juice and cinnamon into a non-stick pan and heat on a medium heat. Cook, stirring continuously, for 2 to 3 minutes. Reduce the heat to medium-low. Cover, simmer and stir occasionally for 6 to 7 minutes. Remove from the heat and immediately stir in the stevia. Set aside to cool.
2. In a small bowl, add the egg whites and beat until stiff peaks form. Fold the egg whites into the rhubarb mixture.
3. Transfer the mixture into serving bowls. Refrigerate to chill before serving.

Strawberry Soufflé

This is a light and delicious dessert which will be a fitting way to your meal. This easy soufflé requires only a few ingredients to assemble.

MAKES: 4 servings
PREPARATION TIME: 10 minutes
COOKING TIME: 10 minutes

10-12 Fresh Strawberries, hulled and sliced
1 tablespoon Applesauce, unsweetened
2 Egg Whites, beaten

Directions:

1. Preheat the oven to 355 degrees F and grease 2 (4-ounce) ramekins.
2. In a blender, add the strawberries and applesauce, and pulse until a smooth puree forms. Transfer the mixture into a bowl. Gently stir in the egg whites.
3. Transfer the mixture into the prepared ramekins and bake for about 10 minutes.

Coconut Macaroons

These coconut macaroons are very easy to assemble and are really delicious. This dessert is a classic and also a kid friendly recipe.

MAKES: 4 servings
PREPARATION TIME: 10 minutes
COOKING TIME: 15 minutes

½ cup Egg Whites
2 tablespoons Coconut Water
Coconut Sugar, to taste
2 cups unsweetened Coconut, shredded

Directions:

1. Preheat the oven to 375 degrees F and line a cookie sheet with baking paper.
2. In a bowl, add the egg whites, coconut water and sugar, and beat until well combined. Stir in the shredded coconut and set aside for 4 to 5 minutes. Make your desired size balls from the coconut mixture. Place the balls onto the prepared cookie sheet in a single layer. Flatten the macaroons slightly with your fingertips.
3. Place the cookie sheet into the oven. Reduce the temperature to 325 degrees F and bake for about 15 minutes.

Citrus Avocado Pudding

This recipe transforms a plain avocado into a healthy dessert. Fresh lime adds a refreshingly tangy touch to this avocado pudding.

MAKES: 2 servings
PREPARATION TIME: 10 minutes

2 large Avocados, peeled, pitted and sliced
Stevia, to taste
2 tablespoons Coconut Oil, melted
2 tablespoons Fresh Lime juice
2 teaspoons Lime Zest, freshly grated

Directions:

1. In a blender, add all of the ingredients and pulse until smooth.
2. Serve immediately.

Lemony Pumpkin Custard

Enjoy a creamy and spiced custard that tastes like a pumpkin pie but is prepared without any fuss.

MAKES: 4 servings
PREPARATION TIME: 15 minutes
COOKING TIME: 30 minutes

1 cup Homemade Pumpkin Puree
2 Egg Whites
¼ cup Almond Milk, unsweetened
¼ cup Applesauce, unsweetened
¼ teaspoon Lemon Zest, freshly grated
½ teaspoon Ground Cinnamon
½ teaspoon Ground Cardamom
½ teaspoon Ground Nutmeg
½ teaspoon Ground Ginger
Pinch of Sea Salt

Directions:

1. Preheat the oven to 350 degrees F and lightly grease 4 (4-ounce) ramekins.
2. In a large bowl, mix together all of the ingredients and beat until smooth. Transfer the mixture into the prepared ramekins. Arrange the ramekins onto a baking sheet.
3. Bake for 25 to 30 minutes.

Mini Fruity Cobblers

This is a great recipe for using seasonal fruits. This delightful summertime treat is prepared with the combination of fresh strawberries and rhubarb.

Makes: 2 servings
PREPARATION TIME: 15 minutes
COOKING TIME: 20 minutes

¾ cup Almond Flour
¼ teaspoon Baking Soda
⅓ teaspoon Ground Cinnamon
Pinch of Sea Salt
¼ cup Almond Milk, unsweetened
3 Egg Whites
4 teaspoons Applesauce, unsweetened
1 cup Coconut Oil, melted
1 cup Fresh Strawberries, hulled and chopped
1 cup Rhubarb, chopped
2 teaspoons Coconut Palm Sugar
3 tablespoons Walnuts, chopped

Directions:

1. Preheat the oven to 350 degrees F and grease 2 (12-ounce) ramekins.
2. In a bowl, mix together the flour, baking soda, ¼ teaspoon of cinnamon and salt. In another bowl, add the milk, egg whites, applesauce and oil, and beat until well

combined.

3. Place the strawberries and rhubarb into the prepared ramekins. Sprinkle with coconut sugar and mix. Top with walnuts. Spread the flour mixture evenly over the fruit, and sprinkle with the remaining cinnamon.

4. Bake for 18 to 20 minutes.

Cinnamon Rice Pudding

This recipe makes a wonderfully delicious and creamy dessert. It requires only a few ingredients for preparation.

Makes: 4 servings
PREPARATION TIME: 15 minutes (plus time to refrigerate)
COOKING TIME: 55 minutes

4½ cups Almond Milk, unsweetened
1 cup Brown Rice
Pinch of Sea Salt
1 teaspoon Ground Cinnamon
Liquid Stevia
¼ cup Walnuts, chopped

Directions:

1. Add the milk, rice and salt into a large pan. Bring to the boil on a medium-high heat. Once the liquid is boiling, reduce the heat and simmer for about 45 minutes, covered. Turn off the heat but keep the pan covered for an extra 10 minutes. Sir in cinnamon and stevia.
2. Transfer the pudding into serving bowls. Cover and refrigerate until fully chilled. Sprinkle with walnuts and serve.

Lime Sorbet

This light and refreshing sorbet will be a great hit on hot summer days. This sorbet has the clean flavor of refreshing lime juice mixed with sweet lime zest.

MAKES: 4 servings
PREPARATION TIME: 10 minutes
(plus ice cream maker and to refrigeration time)

1½ cups Fresh Lime Juice
1 tablespoon Lime Zest, freshly grated
1 teaspoon Liquid Stevia
1½ cups Water

Directions:

1. In a large bowl, mix together all of the ingredients. Cover and refrigerate for about 1 hour. Place the mixture into an ice cream maker and process according to the manufacturer's directions.
2. Transfer the sorbet into an airtight container. Cover and freeze for at least 4 to 5 hours.

Tangy Mint Popsicles

This recipe makes a light and refreshing treat with a combination of some of the freshest summer flavors. These popsicles are really easy to prepare and are so tasty.

MAKES: 4 servings
PREPARATION TIME: 15 minutes (plus time to freeze)
COOKING TIME: 2 minutes

1 teaspoon Lime Zest, freshly grated
1 cup diced Mint Leaves
½ cup Water
1 Cucumber, peeled, seeded and chopped
Liquid Stevia, to taste
⅓ cup Fresh Lime Juice

Directions:

1. In a pan, add the lime zest, mint leaves and water. On a medium heat bring to the boil before removing from the heat. Using a fine sieve, strain the liquid before setting aside to cool slightly.
2. In a food processor, add the cucumber and pulse until chopped very finely. Add the strained water and the remaining ingredients, and pulse until smooth. Transfer the mixture into the Popsicle molds before covering and freezing.

SMOOTHIE RECIPES

Strawberries 'N' Cream Smoothie

Enjoy a lusciously creamy smoothie that has a refreshing zest. Get the good fats from the avocado plus the rich fiber from the combination of all the ingredients.

MAKES: 2 servings
PREPARATION TIME: 5 minutes

½ large Avocado, peeled, pitted and sliced
1 cup Strawberries
1 tablespoon diced Basil Leaves
1½ cups Almond Milk, unsweetened
1 teaspoon Stevia or Coconut Sugar (optional)
½ cup Ice Cubes

Directions:

1. In a blender, add all of the ingredients and pulse until smooth and creamy.
2. Transfer into serving glasses and serve immediately.

Chocolaty Avocado Smoothie

Start off your day by indulging with this super healthy, nutritious and delicious smoothie. With this creamy chocolaty smoothie you'll be full for several hours.

MAKES: 2 servings
PREPARATION TIME: 5 minutes

½ large Avocado, peeled, pitted and sliced
½ tablespoon Stevia
½ cup Blackberries
¼ cup Raw Cacao Powder
2 cups Almond Milk, unsweetened
½ cup Ice Cubes

Directions:

1. In a blender, add all of the ingredients and pulse until smooth and creamy.
2. Transfer into serving glasses and serve immediately.

Spinach Blues Smoothie

This delicious and healthy smoothie will make a nice addition to your breakfast menu. Enjoy those fruits and veggies in the morning when your body needs it most.

MAKES: 2 servings
PREPARATION TIME: 5 minutes

2 tablespoons Goji Berries
1 cup Blueberries, sliced
2 cups Fresh Spinach, torn
1 tablespoon Flax seed Oil
1½ cups Almond Milk, unsweetened
½ cup Ice Cubes

Directions:

1. In a blender, add all of the ingredients and pulse until smooth and creamy.
2. Transfer into serving glasses and serve immediately.

Strawberry Pome Smoothie

This strawberry smoothie is made with pomegranate juice and packs a lot of satisfaction from using the yogurt.

MAKES: 2 servings
PREPARATION TIME: 5 minutes

2 cups Frozen Strawberries
1 cup Plain Yogurt
¾ cup Fresh Pomegranate Juice
¼ cup Water

Directions:

1. In a blender, add all of the ingredients and pulse until smooth and creamy.
2. Transfer into serving glasses and serve immediately.

Mixed Berry Kefir Smoothie

This deliciously strawberry smoothie with kefir is perfect for a quick breakfast. Enjoy a fulfilling glass of simple ingredients.

MAKES: 2 servings
PREPARATION TIME: 5 minutes

1 cup Fresh Strawberries, hulled and sliced
1 cup Fresh Raspberries
2 cups Plain Kefir
½ cup Ice cubes (optional)

Directions:

1. In a blender, add all of the ingredients and pulse until smooth and creamy.
2. Transfer into serving glasses and serve immediately.

Strawberry Quinoa Smoothie

Super healthy quinoa is a great addition to this delicious and refreshing smoothie.

MAKES: 2 servings
PREPARATION TIME: 10 minutes

¼ cup Cashew nuts, soaked and drained
1 cup Quinoa
2 cups Fresh Strawberries, hulled and sliced
1½ cups Water
½ cup Ice Cubes

Directions:

1. In a blender, add the cashew nuts and pulse until chopped very finely. Add the remaining ingredients and pulse until smooth and creamy.
2. Transfer into serving glasses and serve immediately.

Raspberry & Cashew Smoothie

Cashew nuts add a wonderful creaminess to this super easy smoothie. You may also consider substituting the cashews for your favorite nuts in this recipe.

MAKES: 2 servings
PREPARATION TIME: 5 minutes

¼ cup Cashew nuts, soaked and drained
3 cups Frozen Raspberries
2 cups Almond Milk, unsweetened

Directions:

1. In a blender, add the cashew nuts and pulse until chopped very finely. Add the remaining ingredients and pulse until smooth and creamy.
2. Transfer into serving glasses and serve immediately.

Wheatgrass Strawberry Smoothie

This is a classic and delicious smoothie which will be a hit for the whole family. With the health benefits of wheatgrass powder and chia seeds, this makes a unique super food smoothie.

MAKES: 2 servings
PREPARATION TIME: 10 minutes

(plus time to soak the Chia seeds)

1¼ cups Frozen Strawberries or your favorite berries
2 cups Almond Milk, unsweetened
1 tablespoon powdered Wheatgrass
1 tablespoon Chia Seeds (pre-soaked for about 15 minutes)
½ cup Ice Cubes

Directions:

1. In a blender, add all of the ingredients and pulse until smooth and creamy.
2. Transfer into serving glasses and serve immediately.

Strawberry & Kale Protein Smoothie

This protein packed creamy strawberry and kale smoothie is guaranteed to keep you energized all day. With hemp powder in the mix, you'll surely be in for some good nutrition with every sip.

MAKES: 2 servings
PREPARATION TIME: 10 minutes

2 cups Fresh Strawberries
½ cup Fresh Kale, trimmed and chopped
2 tablespoons Hemp Protein Powder
2 cups Almond Milk, unsweetened
1 teaspoon Pumpkin Seed Oil
½ cup Ice Cubes

Directions:

1. In a blender, add all of the ingredients and pulse until smooth and creamy.
2. Transfer into serving glasses and serve immediately.

Spiced Pumpkin Protein Smoothie

This healthy smoothie will quickly replace coffee or tea as your energy booster in the morning. Enjoy this low calorie smoothie which is also very fulfilling.

MAKES: 2 servings
PREPARATION TIME: 10 minutes

½ cup Homemade Pumpkin Puree
½ tablespoon Coconut Oil, melted
1½ cups Almond Milk, unsweetened
3 tablespoons Hemp Protein Powder
¼ teaspoon Ground Nutmeg
¼ teaspoon Ground Cinnamon
¼ teaspoon Ground Ginger
Pinch of Sea Salt
½ cup Ice Cubes

Directions:

1. In a blender, add all of the ingredients and pulse until smooth and creamy.
2. Transfer into serving glasses and serve immediately.

Clean Vera Smoothie

This delicious aloe vera and berry smoothie is full of health promoting benefits. With the added vitamin benefits from the aloe vera plus the rice protein powder, this smoothie turns out to be a nutrition power house.

MAKES: 2 servings
PREPARATION TIME: 10 minutes

1 cup Frozen or Fresh Blueberries
½ cup Fresh Aloe Vera Juice
1½ cups Almond Milk, unsweetened
½ tablespoon Coconut Oil, melted
2 tablespoons Rice Protein Powder

Directions:

1. In a blender, add all of the ingredients and pulse until smooth and creamy.
2. Transfer into serving glasses and serve immediately.

Rich Blueberry Smoothie

This is a delicious blueberry smoothie with the advantages of highly nutritious super food bee pollen.

MAKES: 2 servings
PREPARATION TIME: 10 minutes

2 cups Fresh Blueberries
½ cup Raspberries, peeled, pitted and sliced
1½ cups Almond Milk, unsweetened
1 tablespoon softened Organic Coconut Oil
1 tablespoon Bee Pollen

Directions:

1. In a blender, add all of the ingredients and pulse until smooth and creamy.
2. Transfer into serving glasses and serve immediately.

A LIFETIME WORTH LIVING

There's absolutely no reason why you shouldn't aim to live your best life. Needless to say, the overall lifetime benefits of maintaining a healthy body weight are priceless. It was worth it for me—it will be worth it for you.

As I tell everyone, many people are great starters, but few, really finish what they've started. It will be the few finishers who will really experience an extraordinary life—a lifetime worth living. So, now that you have this cookbook of high protein recipes in your personal library, don't let the book just sit there. Finish what you'd started.

Thanks again for choosing my book. If you find this high protein cookbook to be helpful, I would appreciate if you would let other readers know about it. I now wish you all the best in your pursuit to lose weight, feel better and live a happier life.

Yours in health,
Trisha Myers

CPSIA information can be obtained
at www.ICGtesting.com
Printed in the USA
BVHW031720080919
557867BV00001B/40/P

9 781503 085671